# 49 Gall Bladder Stone Preventing Juice Recipes:

Feed Your Body What it needs to get rid of and Prevent Gall Bladder Stones

By

**Joe Correa CSN**

# COPYRIGHT

© 2017 Live Stronger Faster Inc.

This publication is designed to provide accurate and authoritative information in regard to the subject matter covered. It is sold with the understanding that neither the author nor the publisher is engaged in rendering medical advice. If medical advice or assistance is needed, consult with a doctor. This book is considered a guide and should not be used in any way detrimental to your health. Consult with a physician before starting this nutritional plan to make sure it's right for you.

## ACKNOWLEDGEMENTS

This book is dedicated to my friends and family that have had mild or serious illnesses so that you may find a solution and make the necessary changes in your life.

# 49 Gall Bladder Stone Preventing Juice Recipes:

## Feed Your Body What it needs to get rid of and Prevent Gall Bladder Stones

By

**Joe Correa CSN**

# CONTENTS

## ABOUT THE AUTHOR

After years of Research, I honestly believe in the positive effects that proper nutrition can have over the body and mind. My knowledge and experience has helped me live healthier throughout the years and which I have shared with family and friends. The more you know about eating and drinking healthier, the sooner you will want to change your life and eating habits.

Nutrition is a key part in the process of being healthy and living longer so get started today. The first step is the most important and the most significant.

# INTRODUCTION

49 Gall Bladder Stone Preventing Juice Recipes: Feed Your Body What it needs to get rid of and Prevent Gall Bladder Stones

By Joe Correa CSN

This condition can be easily recognized by constant abdominal pain, especially in the back parts of the abdomen. Depending on the cause, it varies from mild to severe pain that will require hospitalization. But there is one thing in common for this painful condition, it is almost always related to a poor diet and unhealthy eating habits.

The gallbladder is connected to the liver through viaducts. This delicate part of our digestive tract is usually triggered by hormones to release bile when fats reach our duodenum after a heavy meal. This way, gallbladder directly helps the digestion and decomposition of these substances.

However, unhealthy lifestyles and bad eating habits make this process more difficult than ever. Foods that are full of unhealthy fats and highly processed with different artificial substances make this task almost impossible. The logical consequence is a complete blockade of gallbladder ducts and severe inflammation and irritation of the surrounding tissue.

Heartburn, gastritis, and inflammation of the gallbladder are some typical consequences of excessive eating, especially fatty and spicy meals that are extremely hard to digest. To make things worse, these meals are usually combined with unhealthy sodas or alcohol which have a terrible effect on the entire digestive tract. The natural reaction in the body is inflammation of the gallbladder which is often the case with people who have stones in their gallbladder. These stones occur because the body can't excrete enough enzymes that are necessary for digestion. These enzymes are secreted by cells in the stomach and liver and stored in the gallbladder.

Our unhealthy eating habits usually don't create an instant reaction. However, they leave some negative long term effects and contribute to chronical gallbladder problems later in life.

This is why you should start thinking about your gallbladder health right now and do something good for your body. This collection of juices will create very positive and healthy changes in your life, boost your immune system, and help your entire digestive tract work properly. They are easy to make, tasty, and loaded with nutrients that will prevent future serious conditions. Enjoy at least one of these juices every day and stay!

# 49 GALL BLADDER STONE PREVENTING JUICE RECIPES: FEED YOUR BODY WHAT IT NEEDS TO GET RID OF AND PREVENT GALL BLADDER STONES

## 1.    Broccoli Cauliflower Juice

**Ingredients:**

1 cup of broccoli, chopped

1 small cauliflower head

1 large leek

1 cup of fresh kale, torn

1 large green apple, cored

2 oz of water

**Preparation:**

Wash the broccoli and chop into small pieces. Set aside.

Trim off the outer leaves of a cauliflower. Cut into bite-sized pieces and set aside.

Wash the leek and chop into small pieces. Set aside.

Wash the kale thoroughly under cold running water and torn with hands. Set aside.

Wash the apple and remove the core. Cut into bite-sized pieces and set aside.

Now, process broccoli, cauliflower, leek, kale, and apple in a juicer. Transfer to serving glasses and stir in the water.

Add some ice cubes and serve immediately.

Enjoy!

**Nutritional information per serving:** Kcal: 233, Protein: 12.7g, Carbs: 65.7g, Fats: 2.3g

## 2.     Fennel Collard Greens Juice

**Ingredients:**

1 large fennel bulb

1 cup of collard greens

1 large leek

1 cup of mustard greens

1 medium-sized Granny Smith apple, cored

1 large cucumber

**Preparation:**

Wash the fennel bulb and trim off the wilted outer layers. Cut into small chunks and set aside.

Combine collard greens and mustard greens in a large pot. Add 2 cups of hot water and soak for 15 minutes. Drain and set aside.

Wash the leek and roughly chop it. Set aside.

Wash the cucumber and cut into thick slices. Set aside.

Wash the apple and remove the core. Cut into bite-sized pieces and set aside.

Now, process fennel, collard greens, mustard greens, leek, cucumber, and apple in a juicer.

Transfer to serving glasses and add some ice before serving.

Enjoy!

**Nutritional information per serving:** Kcal: 223, Protein: 9.6g, Carbs: 67.9g, Fats: 1.8g

## 3.    Celery Sweet Potato Juice

**Ingredients:**

1 cup of celery, chopped

1 cup of sweet potato, chopped

1 cup of Swiss chard, torn

1 large cucumber

A handful of spinach, torn

2 oz of water

**Preparation:**

Wash the celery and chop into small pieces. Set aside.

Peel the sweet potato and cut into chunks. Fill the measuring cup and reserve the rest for some other juice.

Combine Swiss chard and spinach in a colander. Wash thoroughly under cold running water and torn with hands. Drain and set aside.

Wash the cucumber and cut into thick slices. Set aside.

Now, combine celery, sweet potato, Swiss chard, cucumber, and spinach in a juicer and process until juiced. Transfer to serving glasses and stir in the water.

Refrigerate for 10 minutes before serving.

Enjoy!

**Nutritional information per serving:** Kcal: 156, Protein: 6.3g, Carbs: 43.2g, Fats: 0.8g

## 4.    Artichoke Spring Onion Juice

**Ingredients:**

1 large artichoke

½ cup of spring onions, roughly chopped

1 cup of asparagus, trimmed

1 large cucumber

1 small green apple, cored

1 small ginger root knob, 1-inch

**Preparation:**

Using a sharp knife, trim off the outer leaves of the artichoke. Wash it and cut into small pieces. Set aside.

Place the spring onions in a colander and wash under cold running water. Drain and roughly chop. Set aside.

Wash the asparagus and trim off the woody ends. Chop into small pieces and set aside.

Wash the cucumber and cut into thick slices. Set aside.

Wash the apple and remove the core. Cut into bite-sized pieces and set aside.

Peel the ginger root knob and set aside.

Now, process artichoke, spring onions, asparagus, cucumber, apple, and ginger root in a juicer.

Transfer to serving glasses and add some ice.

Serve immediately.

**Nutritional information per serving:** Kcal: 181, Protein: 11.4g, Carbs: 57.5g, Fats: 1.1g

## 5.     Fuji Banana Juice

**Ingredients:**

1 large Fuji apple, cored

1 large orange

1 large banana

1 medium-sized zucchini

2 oz of water

**Preparation:**

Wash the apple and remove the core. Cut into bite-sized pieces and set aside.

Peel the orange and divide into wedges. Set aside.

Peel the banana and cut into small chunks. Set aside.

Peel the zucchini and cut in half. Scoop out the seeds and cut into small pieces. Set aside.

Now, process apple, orange, banana, and zucchini in a juicer.

Transfer to serving glasses and refrigerate for 15 minutes before serving.

Enjoy!

**Nutritional information per serving:** Kcal: 296, Protein: 6.5g, Carbs: 86.8g, Fats: 1.7g

## 6.    Golden Pineapple Juice

**Ingredients:**

1 cup of pineapple chunks

1 large orange

1 large lemon

1 small Golden Delicious apple, cored

1 cup of celery, chopped

2 oz of water

1 tbsp of honey

**Preparation:**

Cut the top of a pineapple and peel it using a sharp knife. Cut into small chunks. Reserve the rest of the pineapple in a refrigerator for some other juice.

Peel the orange and divide into wedges. Set aside.

Peel the lemon and cut lengthwise in half. Set aside.

Wash the apple and remove the core. Cut into bite-sized pieces and set aside.

Wash the celery and chop into small pieces. Set aside.

Now, combine pineapple, orange, lemon, apple, and celery in a juicer and process until juiced.

Transfer to serving glasses and stir in the water and honey. Add some ice and serve immediately.

Enjoy!

**Nutritional information per serving:** Kcal: 284, Protein: 4.3g, Carbs: 69.2g, Fats: 0.9g

## 7.    Cherry Cantaloupe Juice

**Ingredients:**

1 cup of cherries

1 large green apple, cored

1 cup of cantaloupe, chopped

1 large carrot

2 oz of water

**Preparation:**

Place the cherries in a colander and wash under cold running water. Drain and cut in half. Remove the pits and set aside.

Wash the apple and remove the core. Cut into bite-sized pieces and set aside.

Cut the cantaloupe in half. Scoop out the seeds and cut two large wedges. Peel and chop into chunks. Reserve the rest of the cantaloupe in a refrigerator for some other juice.

Wash the carrot and cut into thick slices. Set aside.

Now, combine cherries, apple, cantaloupe, and carrot in a juicer and process until juiced.

Transfer to serving glasses and stir in the water. Add some ice or refrigerate before serving.

**Nutritional information per serving:** Kcal: 249, Protein: 4.5g, Carbs: 72.3g, Fats: 1.1g

## 8.    Papaya Blueberry Juice

**Ingredients:**

1 small papaya

1 cup of blueberries

1 medium-sized orange

1 cup of watermelon

1 large cucumber

2 oz of water

1 tbsp agave nectar

**Preparation:**

Peel the papaya and cut lengthwise in half. Scoop out the black seeds and flesh using a spoon. Cut into small chunks and set aside.

Wash the blueberries under cold running water. Drain and set aside.

Peel the orange and divide into wedges. Set aside.

Cut the watermelon lengthwise. For one cup, you will need about one large wedge. Peel and cut into chunks.

Remove the seeds and set aside. Reserve the rest of the melon for some other juices.

Wash the cucumber and cut into thick slices. Set aside.

Now, process papaya, blueberries, orange, watermelon, and cucumber in a juicer. Transfer to serving glasses and stir in the water and agave nectar.

Add some ice and serve immediately.

**Nutritional information per serving:** Kcal: 320, Protein: 6g, Carbs: 76.2g, Fats: 1.6g

## 9.    Zucchini Broccoli Juice

**Ingredients:**

1 large zucchini

1 cup of broccoli, chopped

3 large leeks, chopped

1 cup of fresh parsley, torn

A handful of spinach, torn

2 oz of water

**Preparation:**

Peel the zucchini and cut in half. Scoop out the seeds and chop into small pieces. Set aside.

Wash the broccoli and chop into small pieces. Set aside.

Wash the leeks and roughly chop them. Set aside.

Wash the parsley and spinach thoroughly and torn with hands. Set aside.

Now, combine zucchini, broccoli, leeks, parsley, and spinach in a juicer and process until juiced.

Transfer to serving glasses and stir in the water. Add some ice and serve immediately.

Enjoy!

**Nutritional information per serving:** Kcal: 225, Protein: 13.1g, Carbs: 58.7g, Fats: 2.7g

## 10.    Strawberry Cranberry Juice

**Ingredients:**

1 cup of strawberries

1 large Fuji apple, cored

1 cup of cranberries

1 large carrot

1 large lemon

1 large orange

**Preparation:**

Place the strawberries and cranberries in a colander and wash under cold running water. Drain and cut in half. Set aside.

Wash the apple and remove the core. Cut into bite-sized pieces and set aside.

Wash the carrot and cut into thick slices. Set aside.

Peel the lemon cut lengthwise in half. Set aside.

Peel the orange and divide into wedges. Set aside.

Now, process strawberries, apple, cranberries, carrots, lemon, and orange in juicer. Transfer to serving glasses and stir in the water.

Add few ice cubes, or refrigerate for 15 minutes before serving.

**Nutritional information per serving:** Kcal: 268, Protein: 5.6g, Carbs: 89.1g, Fats: 1.6g

## 11.    Beet Lime Juice

**Ingredients:**

3 large beets, trimmed

1 large lime

1 large cucumber

2 celery stalk, chopped

1 small ginger root knob, 1-inch

2 oz of water

**Preparation:**

Wash the beets and trim off the green parts. cut into small pieces and set aside.

Peel the lime and cut lengthwise in half. Set aside.

Wash the cucumber and cut into thick slices. Set aside.

Wash the celery and chop into bite-sized pieces. Set aside.

Peel the ginger root knob and set aside.

Now, combine beets, lime, cucumber, celery, and ginger in a juicer and process until juiced. Transfer to serving glasses and stir in the water.

Refrigerate for 20 minutes before serving.

**Nutritional information per serving:** Kcal: 140, Protein: 6.7g, Carbs: 41.6g, Fats: 0.9g

## 12.    Coconut Blackberry Juice

**Ingredients:**

1 cup of blackberries

1 large orange

1 large yellow apple

1 cup of fresh mint, torn

1 tbsp honey

3 oz coconut water

**Preparation:**

Place the blackberries in a colander and wash under cold running water. Drain and set aside.

Peel the orange and divide into wedges. Set aside.

Wash the apple and remove the core. Cut into bite-sized pieces and set aside.

Place the mint in a bowl and add one cup of lukewarm water. Let it soak for 15 minutes.

Now, combine blackberries, orange, apple, and mint in a juicer and process until juiced.

Transfer to serving glasses and stir in the coconut water and honey. Add some ice and serve immediately.

Enjoy!

**Nutritional information per serving:** Kcal: 287, Protein: 5.3g, Carbs: 88.4g, Fats: 1.5g

## 13.  Avocado Pomegranate Juice

**Ingredients:**

1 cup of avocado

1 cup of pomegranate seeds

1 large cucumber

1 large carrot

¼ tsp of nutmeg

3 oz of water

**Preparation:**

Peel the avocado and cut in half. Remove the pit and cut into small chunks. Set aside.

Cut the top of the pomegranate fruit using a sharp knife. Slice down to each of the white membranes inside of the fruit. Pop the seeds into a bowl and set aside.

Wash the cucumber and carrot. Cut into thick slices and set aside.

Now, combine avocado, pomegranate seeds, cucumber, and carrot in a juicer and process until juiced.

Transfer to serving glasses and stir in the water and nutmeg. Add some ice and serve immediately.

Enjoy!

**Nutritional information per serving:** Kcal: 319, Protein: 7.1g, Carbs: 46.9g, Fats: 23.5g

## 14.    Sweet Potato Tomato Juice

**Ingredients:**

1 cup of sweet potatoes, cubed

2 large Roma tomatoes

1 cup of Swiss chard, torn

1 cup of fresh basil, torn

1 cup of beet greens, torn

¼ tsp of Himalayan salt

2 oz of water

**Preparation:**

Wash the tomatoes and place them in a bowl. Cut into small pieces and reserve the juice while cutting. Set aside.

Peel the sweet potato and cut into cubes. Fill the measuring cup and reserve the rest for some other juice. Set aside.

Combine Swiss chard, basil, and beet greens in a colander and wash under cold running water. Drain and set aside.

Now, process tomatoes, sweet potato, Swiss chard, basil, and beet greens in a juicer.

Transfer to serving glasses and stir in the salt and water.

Refrigerate for 20 minutes before serving.

**Nutritional information per serving:** Kcal: 157, Protein: 7.5g, Carbs: 44.5g, Fats: 1.1g

## 15.  Cantaloupe Squash Juice

**Ingredients:**

1 cup of cantaloupe, chopped

1 cup of butternut squash, chopped

2 large carrots

1 large cucumber

¼ tsp of turmeric, ground

2 oz of water

**Preparation:**

Cut the cantaloupe in half. Scoop out the seeds and flesh. Cut two medium wedges and peel them. Chop into chunks and set aside. Reserve the rest of the cantaloupe in a refrigerator for some other juice.

Peel the butternut squash and remove the seeds using a spoon. Cut into small cubes and reserve the rest of the squash for some other recipe. Wrap in a plastic foil and refrigerate.

Wash the carrots and cucumber and cut into thick slices. Set aside.

Now, combine cantaloupe, butternut squash, carrots, and cucumber in a juicer and process until juiced.

Transfer to serving glasses and stir in the turmeric and water.

Refrigerate for 10 minutes before serving.

Enjoy!

**Nutritional information per serving:** Kcal: 182, Protein: 6g, Carbs: 53.8g, Fats: 1.1g

## 16.    Pineapple Plum Juice

### Ingredients:

1 cup of pineapple chunks

3 large plums, pitted

1 cup of watermelon, chopped

1 large Granny Smith apple, cored

2 oz of coconut water

### Preparation:

Cut the top of a pineapple and peel it using a sharp knife. Cut into small chunks. Reserve the rest of the pineapple in a refrigerator.

Wash the plums and cut in half. Remove the pits and set aside.

Cut the watermelon lengthwise. For one cup, you will need about one large wedge. Peel and cut into chunks. Remove the seeds and set aside. Reserve the rest of the melon for some other juices.

Wash the apple and remove the core. Cut into bite-sized pieces and set aside.

Now, combine pineapple, plums, watermelon, and apple in a juicer and process until juiced.

Transfer to serving glasses and stir in the coconut water.

Add some ice cubes and serve immediately.

Enjoy!

**Nutritional information per serving:** Kcal: 301, Protein: 4.1g, Carbs: 83.7g, Fats: 1.3g

## 17.    Grape Melon Juice

**Ingredients:**

1 cup of green grapes

1 cup of red grapes

1 large Honeydew melon wedge

1 large banana

2 oz of water

**Preparation:**

Combine green and red grapes in a colander and wash under cold running water. Drain and set aside.

Cut the honeydew melon lengthwise in half. Scoop out the seeds using a spoon. Cut one large wedge and peel it. Cut into small chunks and place in a bowl. Wrap the rest of the melon in a plastic foil and refrigerate.

Peel the banana and cut into small chunks. Set aside.

Now, combine grapes, honeydew melon, and banana in a juicer.

Transfer to serving glasses and stir in the water. Add some ice before serving.

Enjoy!

**Nutritional information per serving:** Kcal: 374, Protein: 4.4g, Carbs: 105g, Fats: 1.7g

## 18.    Apple Mint Juice

**Ingredients:**

1 large red apple, cored

1 large carrot

1 large cucumber

1 large orange

1 cup of fresh mint

**Preparation:**

Wash the apple and remove the core. Cut into bite-sized pieces and set aside.

Wash the carrot and cucumber. Cut into thick slices and set aside.

Peel the orange and divide into wedges. Set aside.

Wash the mint and drain. Place it in a bowl and add 1 cup of hot water. Let it soak for 10 minutes. Drain again and set aside.

Now, combine apple, carrots, cucumber, orange, and mint in a juicer and process until juiced. Transfer to serving glasses and add some ice cubes.

Serve immediately.

**Nutritional information per serving:** Kcal: 268, Protein: 6g, Carbs: 79.7g, Fats: 1.5g

## 19.    Cherry Cauliflower Juice

**Ingredients:**

1 cup of cherries

1 small cauliflower head

1 large orange

1 large carrot

1 tbsp of honey

2 oz of water

**Preparation:**

Wash the cherries under cold running water. Drain and cut in half. Remove the pits and set aside.

Trim off the outer leaves of cauliflower. Wash it and cut into small pieces. Set aside.

Peel the orange and divide into wedges. Set aside.

Wash the carrot and cut into thick slices. Set aside.

Now, process cherries, cauliflower, orange, and carrot in a juicer. Transfer to serving glasses and stir in the honey and water.

Add few ice cubes or refrigerate for 10 minutes before serving.

Enjoy!

**Nutritional information per serving:** Kcal: 219, Protein: 9.1g, Carbs: 66.3g, Fats: 1.4g

## 20.  Strawberry Cranberry Juice

**Ingredients:**

1 cup of strawberries, chopped

1 cup of cranberries

1 large green apple, cored

1 cup of fresh kale

1 large cucumber

**Preparation:**

Combine strawberries and cranberries in a colander and wash under cold running water. Drain and cut strawberries in half. Set aside.

Wash the apple and remove the core. Cut into bite-sized pieces and set aside.

Wash the kale thoroughly and drain. Torn with hands and set aside.

Wash the cucumber and cut into thick slices. Set aside.

Now, process strawberries, cranberries, apple, kale, and cucumber. Transfer to serving glasses and add some ice cubes before serving.

Enjoy!

**Nutritional information per serving:** Kcal: 229, Protein: 7.4g, Carbs: 72g, Fats: 1.9g

## 21.    Mango Grapefruit Juice

**Ingredients:**

1 cup of mango chunks

1 large carrot

1 large grapefruit

1 large lemon

1 small pear, cored

2 oz of water

**Preparation:**

Wash the mango and cut into chunks. Fill the measuring cup and reserve the rest for some other juice. Set aside.

Wash the carrot and cut into thick slices. Set aside.

Peel the grapefruit and divide into wedges. Set aside.

Peel the lemon and cut lengthwise in half. Set aside.

Wash the pear and remove the core. Cut into bite-sized pieces and set aside.

Now, process mango, carrot, grapefruit, lemon, and pear in a juicer.

Transfer to serving glasses and add stir in the water. Add some ice cubes or refrigerate for 10 minutes before serving.

Enjoy!

**Nutritional information per serving:** Kcal: 297, Protein: 5.7g, Carbs: 92.7g, Fats: 1.7g

## 22.   Kiwi Avocado Juice

**Ingredients:**

3 large kiwis, peeled

1 cup of avocado chunks

1 large cucumber

1 cup of fresh mint

¼ tsp of vanilla extract

3 oz of water

**Preparation:**

Peel the kiwis and cut lengthwise in half. Set aside.

Peel the avocado and cut in half. Remove the pit and cut into chunks. Reserve the rest for some other juice. Set aside.

Wash the cucumber and cut into thick slices. Set aside.

Wash the mint thoroughly under cold running water. Set aside.

Now, combine kiwis, avocado, cucumber, and mint in a juicer and process until juiced. Transfer to serving glasses and stir in the water and vanilla extract.

Add some ice and serve immediately.

Enjoy!

**Nutritional information per serving:** Kcal: 351, Protein: 8.3g, Carbs: 57.8g, Fats: 23.6g

## 23.    Artichoke Pea Juice

**Ingredients:**

1 large artichoke

1 cup of green peas

1 cup of collard greens, torn

1 medium-sized apple, cored

1 cup of carrots, sliced

¼ tsp of Himalayan salt

2 oz of water

**Preparation:**

Using a sharp knife, trim off the outer layers of the artichoke. Wash it and cut into bite-sized pieces. Set aside.

Place the green peas in a colander and wash under cold running water. Drain and set aside.

Wash the collard greens thoroughly and torn with hands. Set aside.

Wash the carrots and slice into thin slices. Fill the measuring cup and reserve the rest for some other juice. Set aside.

Now, process artichoke, green peas, collard greens, and carrots in a juicer. Transfer to serving glasses and refrigerate for 10 minutes before serving.

**Nutritional information per serving:** Kcal: 250, Protein: 16.2g, Carbs: 74.9g, Fats: 1.7g

## 24.    Green Bean Kale Juice

**Ingredients:**

1 cup of green beans, chopped

1 cup of fresh kale, torn

1 large apple, cored

1 cup of red leaf lettuce, torn

1 large lime

1 large red bell pepper

1 small ginger root knob, 1-inch

3 oz of water

**Preparation:**

Wash the green beans and chop into bite-sized pieces. Set aside.

Combine kale and red leaf lettuce in a colander and wash thoroughly under cold running water. Torn with hands and set aside.

Wash the apple and remove the core. Cut into bite-sized pieces and set aside.

Peel the lime and cut lengthwise in half. Set aside.

Wash the red bell pepper and cut in half. Remove the seeds and chop into small pieces. Set aside.

Peel the ginger root knob and set aside.

Now, process green beans, kale, red leaf lettuce, apple, lime, red bell pepper, and ginger root in a juicer.

Transfer to serving glasses and stir in the water. Add some ice and serve immediately.

**Nutritional information per serving:** Kcal: 194, Protein: 7.1g, Carbs: 52.9g, Fats: 1.7g

## 25.   Cantaloupe Apple Juice

**Ingredients:**

2 cups of cantaloupe, chopped

1 large Fuji apple, cored

1 large carrot

1 large orange

1 large lemon

**Preparation:**

Cut the cantaloupe in half. Scoop out the seeds and flesh. You will need about four large wedges for two cups. Cut and peel them. Chop into chunks and set aside. Reserve the rest of the cantaloupe in a refrigerator.

Wash the apple and remove the core. Cut into bite-sized pieces and set aside.

Peel the orange and lemon. Divide orange into wedges and cut lemon lengthwise in half. Set aside.

Now, process cantaloupe, apple, carrot, orange, and lemon in a juicer.

Transfer to serving glasses and add few ice cubes before serving.

**Nutritional information per serving:** Kcal: 291, Protein: 6.5g, Carbs: 87.4g, Fats: 1.5g

## 26.    Asparagus Zucchini Juice

**Ingredients:**

1 cup of asparagus, trimmed

1 large zucchini

1 cup of collard greens

1 large lemon

2 large leeks

¼ tsp of Himalayan salt

2 oz of water

**Preparation:**

Wash the asparagus and trim off the woody ends. Cut into small pieces, about 1-inch. Set aside.

Peel the zucchini and cut in half. Scrape out the seeds and cut into chunks. Set aside.

Wash the collard greens thoroughly under cold running water. Drain and torn with hands. Set aside.

Peel the lemon and cut lengthwise in half. Set aside.

Wash the leeks and roughly chop it. Set aside.

Now, combine asparagus, zucchini, collard greens, lemon, and leeks in a juicer and process until juiced.

Transfer to serving glasses and stir in the salt and water.

Refrigerate for 15 minutes before serving.

**Nutritional information per serving:** Kcal: 171, Protein: 11.2g, Carbs: 47.8g, Fats: 2.1g

## 27.    Celery Carrot Juice

**Ingredients:**

2 cups of celery, chopped

3 large carrots

1 large cucumber

1 cup of sweet potatoes, cubed

1 small ginger root knob, 1-inch

**Preparation:**

Wash the celery and cut into small pieces. Set aside.

Wash the carrots and cucumber. Cut into thick slices and set aside.

Peel the sweet potato and cut into cubes. Fill the measuring cup and reserve the rest for some other juice. Set aside.

Peel the ginger knob and set aside.

Now, process celery, carrots, cucumber, potatoes, and ginger in a juicer.

Transfer to serving glasses and refrigerate for 10 minutes before serving.

Enjoy!

**Nutritional information per serving:** Kcal: 228, Protein: 7.6g, Carbs: 65.4g, Fats: 1.3g

## 28.    Pineapple Broccoli Juice

**Ingredients:**

1 cup of pineapple chunks

1 cup of broccoli

2 cups of green grapes

1 large Granny Smith apple

2 oz of coconut water

1 tsp of honey

**Preparation:**

Cut the top of a pineapple and peel it using a sharp knife. Cut into small chunks. Reserve the rest of the pineapple in a refrigerator.

Wash the broccoli and cut into small pieces. Set aside.

Place the grapes in a colander and wash under cold running water. Drain and set aside.

Wash the apple and remove the core. Cut into bite-sized pieces and set aside.

Now, combine pineapple chunks, broccoli, grapes, and apple in a juicer and process until juiced.

Transfer to serving glasses and stir in the coconut water and honey. Stir well and add few ice cubes before serving.

Enjoy!

**Nutritional information per serving:** Kcal: 358, Protein: 5.5g, Carbs: 97.3g, Fats: 1.6g

## 29.    Squash Pomegranate Juice

**Ingredients:**

2 cups of butternut squash, chopped

1 cup of pomegranate seeds

1 large lemon

1 large orange

1 cup of celery chopped

2 oz of water

**Preparation:**

Peel the butternut squash and remove the seeds using a spoon. Cut into small cubes and reserve the rest of the squash for some other recipe. Wrap in a plastic foil and refrigerate.

Cut the top of the pomegranate fruit using a sharp knife. Slice down to each of the white membranes inside of the fruit. Pop the seeds into a medium bowl.

Peel the lemon and orange. Divide orange into wedges and cut lemon lengthwise in half. Set aside.

Wash the celery and chop into small pieces. Set aside.

Now, combine butternut squash, pomegranate seeds, lemon, orange, and celery in a juicer and process until juiced.

Transfer to serving glasses and stir in the water. Add few ice cubes and serve immediately.

Enjoy!

**Nutritional information per serving:** Kcal: 251, Protein: 7.3g, Carbs: 79g, Fats: 1.8g

## 30. Collard Greens Carrot Juice

**Ingredients:**

3 cups of collard greens, torn

2 large carrots

1 medium-sized sweet potato, cubed

1 large cucumber

1 cup of fresh basil, torn

**Preparation:**

Combine collard greens and basil in a colander. Wash under cold running water and drain. Torn with hands and set aside.

Wash the carrots and cucumber and cut into thick slices. Set aside.

Peel the sweet potato and chop into cubes. Set aside.

Now, process collard greens, carrots, sweet potato, cucumber, and basil in a juicer. Transfer to serving glasses and refigerate for 15 minutes or add some ice and serve immediately.

**Nutritional information per serving:** Kcal: 201, Protein: 9.3g, Carbs: 57.3g, Fats: 1.5g

## 31.   Grapefruit Plum Juice

**Ingredients:**

1 large grapefruit

1 cup of mango, chopped

3 large plums, pitted

1 medium-sized green apple, cored

2 oz of coconut water

A few mint leaves

**Preparation:**

Peel the grapefruit and divide into wedges. Set aside.

Wash the mango and cut into chunks. Fill the measuring cup and refrigerate the rest for some other juice. Set aside.

Wash the plums and cut in half. Remove the pits and chop into small pieces. Set aside.

Wash the apple and remove the core. Cut into bite-sized pieces and set aside.

Now, process grapefruit, mango, plums, and apple in a juicer. Transfer to serving glasses and stir in the coconut water.

Add few ice cubes and garnish with mint.

Serve immediately.

**Nutritional information per serving:** Kcal: 211, Protein: 9.3g, Carbs: 59.3g, Fats: 1.5g

## 32.    Pear Kiwi Juice

**Ingredients:**

2 large pears, cored

1 large kiwi

1 large cucumber

1 large carrot

2 oz of water

1 tbsp of liquid honey

**Preparation:**

Wash the pears and remove the core. Cut into bite-sized pieces and set aside.

Peel the kiwi and cut lengthwise in half. Set aside.

Wash the carrot and cucumber and cut into thick slices. Set aside.

Now, combine pears, kiwi, carrot, and cucumber in a juicer and process until juiced. Transfer to serving glasses and add some ice cubes before serving.

Enjoy!

**Nutritional information per serving:** Kcal: 361, Protein: 5.1g, Carbs: 109g, Fats: 1.5g

## 33. Citrus Asparagus Juice

**Ingredients:**

1 cup of asparagus, trimmed

1 large orange

1 cup of green grapes

1 large lemon

1 large lime

3 oz of water

**Preparation:**

Wash the asparagus and trim off the woody ends. Cut into 1-inch pieces and set aside.

Peel the orange and divide into wedges. Set aside.

Wash the green grapes under cold running water. Drain water and set aside.

Peel the lemon and lime and cut lengthwise in half. Set aside.

Now, process asparagus, orange, grapes, lemon, and lime in a juicer.

Transfer to serving glasses and stir in the water. Add some ice and serve immediately.

Enjoy!

**Nutritional information per serving:** Kcal: 361, Protein: 5.1g, Carbs: 109g, Fats: 1.5g

## 34.   Brussels Sprouts Turnip Juice

**Ingredients:**

2 cups of Brussels sprouts, halved

1 cup of turnip greens, torn

3 large radishes, trimmed

3 large leeks, chopped

1 large cucumber

2 oz of water

**Preparation:**

Wash the Brussels sprouts and remove the outer layers. Cut in half and set aside.

Wash the turnip greens under cold running water. Drain and torn with hands. Set aside.

Wash the radishes and trim off the green parts. Set aside.

Wash the leeks and cut into bite-sized pieces. Set aside.

Wash the cucumber and cut into thick slices. Set aside.

Now, combine Brussels sprouts, turnip greens, radishes, leeks, and cucumber in a juicer and process until juiced. Transfer to serving glasses and stir in the water.

Refrigerate for 10 minutes before serving.

**Nutritional information per serving:** Kcal: 247, Protein: 12.9g, Carbs: 69.3g, Fats: 1.8g

## 35.    Purple Cabbage Mango Juice

**Ingredients:**

2 large Fuji apples, cored

1 cup of purple cabbage, torn

1 cup of mango, chopped

1 cup of fresh basil, torn

1 small carrot

¼ tsp of ginger, ground

**Preparation:**

Wash the apples and remove the core. Cut into bite-sized pieces and set aside.

Combine cabbage and basil in a colander. Wash thoroughly under cold running water and torn with hands. Set aside.

Wash the mango and cut into small chunks. Fill the measuring cup and reserve the rest for some other juice. Set aside.

Wash the carrot and cut into thick slices. Set aside.

Now, process apples, purple cabbage, mango, basil, and carrots in a juicer. Transfer to serving glasses and stir in ginger.

Refrigerate for about 10-15 minutes before serving.

**Nutritional information per serving:** Kcal: 319, Protein: 5.6g, Carbs: 92.7g, Fats: 1.8g

## 36. Tomato Cauliflower Juice

**Ingredients:**

2 medium-sized tomatoes

1 large red bell pepper, chopped

1 cup of cauliflower

1 large lime

3 oz of water

1 tsp of fresh rosemary, finely chopped

**Preparation:**

Wash the tomatoes and place them in a bowl. Cut into quarters and reserve the juice while cutting. Set aside.

Wash the bell pepper and cut in half. Remove the seeds and chop into small slices. Set aside.

Trim off the outer leaves of cauliflower. Wash it and cut into small pieces. Reserve the rest in the refrigerator.

Peel the lime and cut lengthwise in half. Set aside.

Now, combine tomatoes, red bell pepper, cauliflower, and lime in a juicer and process until juiced.

Transfer to serving glasses and stir in the reserved tomato juice and water. Sprinkle with fresh rosemary and refrigerate for 10 minutes before serving.

Enjoy!

**Nutritional information per serving:** Kcal: 98, Protein: 6g, Carbs: 28.5g, Fats: 1.3g

## 37.  Blueberry Banana Juice

**Ingredients:**

2 cups of blueberries

1 large banana

1 small Golden Delicious apple, cored

1 large cucumber

2 oz of water

Preparation:

Place the blueberries in a colander and wash under cold running water. Drain and set aside.

Peel the banana and cut into small chunks. Set aside.

Wash the apple and remove the core. Cut into bite-sized pieces and set aside.

Wash the cucumber and cut into thick slices. Set aside.

Now, process blueberries, banana, apple, and cucumber in a juicer. Transfer to serving glasses and add some ice before serving.

Enjoy!

**Nutritional information per serving:** Kcal: 348, Protein: 6g, Carbs: 102g, Fats: 1.9g

## 38.    Romaine Lettuce Artichoke Juice

**Ingredients:**

3 cups of Romaine lettuce

1 cup of spinach, torn

1 medium-sized artichoke

1 large Honeydew melon wedge

1 small green apple, cored

2 large carrots

2 oz of water

**Preparation:**

Wash the lettuce and spinach thoroughly under cold running water and set aside.

Trim off the outer leaves of the artichoke using a sharp knife. Cut into small pieces and set aside.

Cut the honeydew melon lengthwise in half. Scoop out the seeds using a spoon. Cut one large wedge and peel them. Cut into small chunks and fill the measuring cup. Wrap the rest of the melon in a plastic foil and refrigerate.

Wash the apple and remove the core. Cut into bite-sized pieces and set aside.

Wash the carrots and cut into thick slices. Set aside.

Now, combine lettuce, artichoke, honeydew melon, apple, and carrots in a juicer and process until juiced. Transfer to serving glasses and stir in the water.

Add some ice and serve immediately.

**Nutritional information per serving:** Kcal: 213, Protein: 9.6g, Carbs: 67.1g, Fats: 1.5g

## 39.    Cantaloupe Squash Juice

**Ingredients:**

2 cups of cantaloupe

1 cup of crookneck squash, chopped

1 cup of raspberries

1 large apricot

1 large kiwi

**Preparation:**

Cut the cantaloupe in half. Scoop out the seeds and flesh. Cut two wedges and peel them. Chop into chunks and set aside. Reserve the rest of the cantaloupe in a refrigerator.

Wash the crookneck squash and cut in half. Scoop out the seeds using a spoon. Cut into small chunks and set aside. Reserve the rest for another juice.

Wash the raspberries under cold running water and set aside.

Wash the apricot and cut in half. Remove the pit and cut into chunks. Set aside.

Peel the kiwi and cut lengthwise in half. Set aside.

Now, process cantaloupe, crookneck squash, raspberries, apricots, and kiwi in a juicer.

Transfer to serving glasses and add some ice before serving.

Enjoy!

**Nutritional information per serving:** Kcal: 193, Protein: 6.6g, Carbs: 59.1g, Fats: 2.3g

## 40.  Parsnip Pepper Juice

**Ingredients:**

2 cups of parsnips

1 large green bell pepper

1 cup of Swiss chard, torn

1 large cucumber

1 ginger root knob, 1-inch

2 oz of water

**Preparation:**

Wash the parsnips and trim off the green parts. Cut into bite-sized pieces and set aside.

Wash the bell pepper and cut into half. Remove the seeds and cut into small slices. Set aside.

Wash the Swiss chard thoroughly and torn with hands. Set aside.

Peel the ginger and set aside.

Now, process parsnips, bell pepper, Swiss chard, cucumber, and ginger knob in a juicer.

Transfer to serving glasses and stir in the water.

Add some ice and serve immediately.

Enjoy!

**Nutritional information per serving:** Kcal: 219, Protein: 7.3g, Carbs: 68.8g, Fats: 1.5g

## 41.    Peach Cranberry Juice

### Ingredients:

1 large peach

1 cup of cranberries

2 small Granny Smith apples

1 cup of grapes

2 oz of water

### Preparation:

Wash the peach and cut in half. Remove the pit and cut into chunks. Set aside.

Wash the cranberries and grapes under cold running water and set aside.

Wash the apples and remove the core. Cut into bite-sized pieces and set aside.

Now, combine peach, cranberries, apples, and grapes in a juicer and process until juiced. Transfer to serving glasses and add some ice.

Serve immediately.

**Nutritional information per serving:** Kcal: 284, Protein: 2.8g, Carbs: 85g, Fats: 1.4g

## 42.   Papaya Grapefruit Juice

**Ingredients:**

1 cup of papaya, chopped

1 large grapefruit

1 large cucumber

1 small green apple

2 oz of coconut water

**Preparation:**

Peel the papaya and cut lengthwise in half. Scoop out the black seeds and flesh using a spoon. Cut into small chunks and fill the measuring cup. Reserve the rest for some other juice. Set aside.

Peel the grapefruit and divide into wedges. Set aside.

Wash the cucumber and cut into thick slices. Set aside.

Wash the apple and remove the core. Cut into bite-sized pieces and set aside.

Now, process papaya, grapefruit, cucumber, and apple in a juicer. Transfer to serving glasses and stir in the coconut water.

Add few ice cubes and serve immediately.

**Nutritional information per serving:** Kcal: 246, Protein: 5.1g, Carbs: 72.4g, Fats: 1.3g

### 43.    Pomegranate Strawberry Juice

**Ingredients:**

1 cup of pomegranate seeds

1 cup of strawberries

1 large green apple

1 large orange

A handful of spinach

2 oz of water

**Preparation:**

Cut the top of the pomegranate fruit using a sharp knife. Slice down to each of the white membranes inside of the fruit. Pop the seeds into a medium bowl.

Wash the strawberries and cut in half. Set aside.

Wash the apple and remove the core. Cut into bite-sized pieces and set aside.

Wash the spinach thoroughly and torn with hands. Set aside.

Peel the orange and divide into wedges. Set aside.

Now, process pomegranate seeds, strawberries, apple, spinach, and orange in a juicer. Transfer to serving glasses and stir in the water.

Refrigerate for 15 minutes before serving.

**Nutritional information per serving:** Kcal: 266, Protein: 6.1g, Carbs: 80.8g, Fats: 2.2g

## 44.    Green Bean Zucchini Juice

**Ingredients:**

1 cup of green beans, chopped

1 large zucchini, chopped

1 cup of sweet potatoes

1 large lemon

¼ tsp of Himalayan salt

2 oz of water

**Preparation:**

Wash the green beans and cut into 1-inch pieces. Set aside.

Peel the zucchini and cut in half. Scoop out the seeds and cut into chunks. Set aside.

Peel the sweet potatoes and cut into small cubes. Fill the measuring cup and reserve the rest for some other juice. Set aside.

Peel the lemon and cut lengthwise in half. Set aside.

Now, process green beans, zucchini, sweet potatoes, and lemon in a juicer and stir in the water.

Add some ice or refrigerate before serving.

Enjoy!

**Nutritional information per serving:** Kcal: 171, Protein: 7.6g, Carbs: 46g, Fats: 1.3g

## 45.    Kale Cucumber Juice

**Ingredients:**

3 cups of fresh kale, torn

1 large cucumber

1 large plum

1 small green apple, cored

1 tbsp of honey

2 oz of water

**Preparation:**

Wash the kale thoroughly under cold running water. Drain and set aside.

Wash the cucumber and cut into thick slices. Set aside.

Wash the plum and cut in half. Remove the pit and cut into small pieces. Set aside.

Wash the apple and remove the core. Cut into bite-sized pieces and set aside.

Now, combine kale, cucumber, plum, and apple in a juicer and process until juiced. Transfer to serving glasses and stir in the honey and water.

Enjoy!

**Nutritional information per serving:** Kcal: 262, Protein: 11.6g, Carbs: 72.6g, Fats: 2.6g

## 46.    Mango Beet Juice

**Ingredients:**

1 cup of mango, chopped

3 large beets, trimmed

1 small apple, cored

1 cup of broccoli

3 oz of coconut water

**Preparation:**

Wash the mango and cut into chunks. Fill the measuring cup and reserve the rest for some other juice. Set aside.

Wash the beets and trim off the green parts. Cut into small pieces and set aside.

Wash the apple and remove the core. Cut into bite-sized pieces and set aside.

Wash the broccoli and cut into small pieces. Set aside.

Now, combine mango, beets, apple, and broccoli in a juicer and process until juiced.

Transfer to serving glasses and add some ice before serving.

Enjoy!

**Nutritional information per serving:** Kcal: 260, Protein: 8.2g, Carbs: 71.8g, Fats: 1.6g

## 47.    Cherry Apple Juice

**Ingredients:**

1 cup of cherries

1 small apple, cored

1 large carrot

1 large orange

1 large lemon

2 oz of water

**Preparation:**

Wash the cherries thoroughly and cut in half. Remove the pits and set aside.

Wash the apple and remove the core. Cut into bite-sized pieces and set aside.

Wash the carrot and cut into thick slices. Set aside.

Peel the lemon and orange. Cut lemon lengthwise in half and divide orange into wedges. Set aside.

Now, combine cherries, apple, carrot, lemon, and orange in a juicer and process until juiced. Transfer to serving glasses and add some ice before serving.

Enjoy!

**Nutritional information per serving:** Kcal: 253, Protein: 5.3g, Carbs: 78.2g, Fats: 1.1g

## 48.    Pumpkin Pineapple Juice

**Ingredients:**

1 cup of pumpkin, chopped

1 cup of apricot, chopped

1 cup of pineapple chunks

1 medium-sized zucchini

1 medium-sized apple, cored

2 oz of water

**Preparation:**

Peel the pumpkin and cut in half. Scoop out the seeds using a spoon. Cut one large wedge and peel it. Cut into small chunks and set aside. Reserve the rest for later.

Wash the apricots and cut in half. Remove the pits and cut into pieces. Fill the measuring cup and reserve the rest for some other juice. Set aside.

Cut the top of a pineapple and peel it using a sharp knife. Cut into small chunks. Reserve the rest of the pineapple in a refrigerator.

Peel the zucchini and cut in half. Scoop out the seeds and cut into cubes. Set aside.

Wash the apple and remove the core. Cut into bite-sized pieces and set aside.

Now, process pumpkin, apricots, pineapple, zucchini, and apple in a juicer.

Transfer to serving glasses and stir in the water. Add some ice and serve immediately.

**Nutritional information per serving:** Kcal: 272, Protein: 7.2g, Carbs: 76.6g, Fats: 1.8g

## 49. Kiwi Watermelon Juice

**Ingredients:**

3 large kiwis

2 cups of watermelon, chopped

3 large strawberries, halved

1 large orange

2 oz of coconut water

**Preparation:**

Peel the kiwis and cut lengthwise in half. Set aside.

Cut the watermelon lengthwise. For two cups, you will need about two large wedges. Peel and cut into chunks. Remove the seeds and set aside. Reserve the rest of the melon for some other juices.

Wash the strawberries and cut in half. Set aside.

Peel the orange and divide into wedges. Set aside.

Now, combine kiwis, watermelon, strawberries, and orange in a juicer and process until juiced. Transfer to serving glasses and stir in the coconut water.

Add some ice cubes and serve immediately.

**Nutritional information per serving:** Kcal: 280, Protein: 6.3g, Carbs: 81.1g, Fats: 1.9g

## ADDITIONAL TITLES FROM THIS AUTHOR

70 Effective Meal Recipes to Prevent and Solve Being Overweight: Burn Fat Fast by Using Proper Dieting and Smart Nutrition

By

Joe Correa CSN

48 Acne Solving Meal Recipes: The Fast and Natural Path to Fixing Your Acne Problems in Less Than 10 Days!

By

Joe Correa CSN

41 Alzheimer's Preventing Meal Recipes: Reduce or Eliminate Your Alzheimer's Condition in 30 Days or Less!

By

Joe Correa CSN

70 Effective Breast Cancer Meal Recipes: Prevent and Fight Breast Cancer with Smart Nutrition and Powerful Foods

By

Joe Correa CSN